Looking Anxiety in the Face

Looking Anxiety in the Face

Wisdom for All Who Worry

HERBERT BROKERING

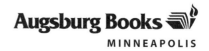

Augsburg Books

MINNEAPOLIS

Looking Anxiety in the Face
Wisdom for All Who Worry

Living Well Series

Cover art: © Dougal Waters/Getty Images.
Cover design: Laurie Ingram
Interior design: PerfecType, Nashville, TN

Library of Congress Cataloging-in-Publication Data

Brokering, Herbert, 1926-
    Looking anxiety in the face : wisdom for all who worry / Herbert Brokering.
        p. cm. — (Living well series)
    ISBN 978-0-8066-7059-1 (alk. paper)
    1. Anxiety—Religious aspects—Christianity. 2. Worry—Religious aspects—Christianity. I. Title.
    BV4908.5.B745 2009
    242'.4—dc22
                                                    2009011773

Manufactured in the U.S.A.

13   12   11   10   09   1   2   3   4   5   6   7   8   9   10

Contents

Emotions have their own energy.
It is data, power, fuel for a task
for decisions to be made by me.
For what shall I spend the emotion?
That is what I ask . . . what I ask.

Anxiety has the power of a raging sea
And will lift a ship to the tip of a wave,
Can break a good life on the rock of a shore.
Or surge in my body to make me more brave.
In a storm I can lift an anchor and far more
And a rock . . . and far more, and far more.

- 1 -

Anxiety
An Exploration

Come gracious Spirit, heavenly dove,
With light and comfort from above.
Come be our guardian and our guide;
O'er every thought and step preside.[1]

I will be the first to admit that I am no stranger to worry. For most of my life I have been an anxious person, fearful and uncertain, knowing dread. So many times I have watched as anxiety gathers like black rain clouds over the prairie, knowing that the storm is breaking, knowing that I am going to get rained on, going to get very wet.

Anxious thoughts, anxious feelings have troubled many nights, constricted many days. Worries and fears, sometimes real, often imagined, have shut doors that should be propped open, drawn boundaries where there should be none, and given rise to a strange loneliness that strangely resists the love and care of loving and caring people all around me.

There are so many triggers of wearisome worry—events, memories, anticipations—it's hard to keep track of them all. Which is one of the reasons for this little book. It helps to name the triggers of anxiety; it takes some of their power away; it creates a space to think, to feel, to trust the "light and comfort from above."

So, yes, I am an anxious person. But I am also a curious person. I want to know, to understand the worries that gather over my head, and in my head and heart and soul. Which is another reason for this little book. It helps me—and I hope it will help you—to look the many signs, sides, and faces of anxiety in the face and see what can be seen, learn what can be learned, and, in the seeing and the learning, grow a bit in understanding and accepting myself—and God.

Some things help some times—not every time, but some times. With anxiety as a traveling companion these many years, I have had plenty of opportunities to learn what—at times—keeps my willful escort at arm's length. Maybe what has helped me at times will help you at times. That is my hope, and another reason for writing this little book.

So, I am an anxious person and a curious person. I am also a person who has always—as have we all—lived in a remarkable network of relationships: family, friends, co-workers and collaborators, and chance acquaintances who have encouraged and inspired. Which is to say that anxiety has not been my only companion these many years. One cannot imagine the journey without all these others. This little book is a tip of the hat in memory and in thanks to them, and an encouragement to you to tip your own hat to those who have accompanied you.

Anxious, curious, networked—that describes me well, but one descriptor is lacking: I am also a person of faith. I grew up in the faith of my mother and father and have never grown away from it—although it is mine now and in some ways larger. In thrall to anxiety, I have at times experienced what seemed the silence and absence of God, but strangely enough, in the throes of anxiety, I have also heard the voice of God in song and in sighing, in words of comfort and cheer, in birds and crickets and leaves blowing in a spring breeze, in baby's crying and mother's cooing, in the sounds of honest work. Faith has kept me hopeful:

Lord of all hopefulness, Lord of all joy,
Whose trust, ever childlike, no cares could destroy:
Be there at our waking, and give us, we pray,
Your bliss in our hearts, Lord, at the break of the day.

Lord of all eagerness, Lord of all faith,
Whose strong hands were skilled at the plane and the lathe:
Be there at our labors, and give us, we pray,
Your strength in our hearts, Lord, at the noon of the day.

Lord of all kindliness, Lord of all grace,
Your hands swift to welcome, your arms to embrace:
Be there at our homing, and give us, we pray,
Your love in our hearts, Lord, at the eve of the day.

Lord of all gentleness, Lord of all calm,
Whose voice is contentment, whose presence is balm:
Be there at our sleeping, and give us, we pray,
Your peace in our hearts, Lord, at the end of the day.[2]

I am an anxious, curious, networked, person of faith who, in the words of an ancient poet, is "fearfully and wonderfully made" (Psalm 139:14). This little book is a celebration of me, anxiety and all, and hopefully, a celebration of you, anxiety and all.

— An idea to practice —

As you read through this book, let it be a window on your own experiences of anxiety, curiosity, relationships, and faith. Write down in a notebook what of my experience resonates with your own experience, as well as what in your experience is different from mine. We are both similar and unique—reflecting on our similarities can open a window on our uniqueness.

- 2 -

Anxiety

Reality

Just as I am though tossed about,
With many a conflict, many a doubt
Fightings and fears, within, without,
O Lamb of God, I come, I come.[3]

My eyes are shut, and I stare at what I feel and think. I am anxious about something that is not present. It feels bigger than life but is not real. My eyes stay shut so I can study the emotion, figure it out, give it a name. I hope to comprehend so it will disappear. The haunting feeling does not go away and plays tag with other emotions as unreal and again bigger than life.

O Lord, show me a dove. Let me see the wounds in your hands and in your side. I am Thomas. I have eyes to see, and ears to hear and a voice to speak. Take me to a tree. I need to touch the balm in Gilead.

My eyes are shut and I remember from the past the voice of someone: "Open your eyes; look, find something real, get in touch with the real world." I am near a window and I see the limb of a blooming apple tree. My eyes are fixed on the green leaves and the closing white blossoms. It is early night. Good, I am feeling a difference. Alas. My eyes slowly close and I am again lost in a fog—not outside my window, nor as happy, but roaming inside myself, one of deep emotion.

This spring is not the first time I am this way. I know this feeling in any season, winter and fall and beautiful summer. Anxiety is no respecter of seasons. It is spring, and I want my emotions to match the joy outside the window. It occurs to me that the window is in the way. The tree is like a painting. I open the window and feel the fresh air. This is better. I smell the blossoms and hear the soft wind in leaves. How long will I stay by the open window to be in touch with reality? I focus on the tree. Will I be at the window all night? I tell myself I do not need a new worry; this is an old voice I hear. Quietly I am rested and captured by the tree. I stay, breathing the wind. This is a better way to live. I hear the leaves. I have found a song in the branches, for this time. The song and dancing branch were there before; I have found a moment of reality again. How long will peace last? I need it for this hour, and then again.

Now it is another night; the evening was just right for sleeping; I am awake. The open window is not enough. There was still the screen, a wire scrim. I go out and touch the tree. The wind touches me from several directions. I am surrounded by reality. My attention is on the valley and crab apples and night sky. I stand there as reality absorbs me like a sacred icon.

I would go back inside soon. All this makes night a friend and an apple tree a gentle mother. Night reaches out to give herself to me.

Take the bread, break it, share it, eat it. Be whole. Touch the branch, see the leaves move, watch the wind and become real. Be whole. The wind is my breath. Wind of God, save me. Tree of God, save me. Find salvation in a tree, in hay, in a drink, in another, on the water, through breaking bread.

The ashes of baby Henry are under a tree. The seasons of the maple keep me in reality. I savor the tree; Henry is fine.

MAPLE TREE SONG

The maple tree is silent,
the snow upon each stem;
there is a sleep so quiet
we know not why or when.

The maple tree is silent,
gold leaves are 'neath the snow
and if we watch the maple,
we know where winters go.

The maple tree is silent,
it is more still than still;
the leaves will soon be budding,
I know they will, they will.[4]

– An idea to practice –

When you feel anxious "about something that is not present," try to ground yourself in reality by drawing your attention deeply into the present moment. A therapist can teach you calming exercises to relax or release tension. These natural body exercises will draw your attention to your body away from inner thoughts that can play tricks. Body motions can help you to focus on the real world. Be aware of what is concretely real around you: feel textures, touch trees and stones; be aware of the touch of the wind or the sun or the cold; smell flowers, catch the scent of a loved one, sniff the aromas of the kitchen or the barn, an apple orchard or hayfield; taste good food, chew and drink slowly, savoring the meal or midnight snack; see colors, lose yourself in their many shades and hues and patterns; notice shapes, feel roundness and squareness. Anxiety draws power from that which is not real, from the rehashed past and rehearsed future. Anxiety loses power in the concrete immediacy of the present moment.

- 3 -

Anxiety
Breath

Breathe on me, breath of God;
So shall I never die,
But live with you the perfect life
Of your eternity.[5]

I know the hymn by heart, and then, while praying, the thought comes, and I fear again: "What if I ran out of breath?" When I have this feeling, I struggle; I struggle with the thought and with breathing. I sometimes struggle like a drowning person.

The pattern is almost always the same. Life and emotion and breath go on unnoticed. I am on automatic, and I need do nothing to keep life going. And then suddenly it dawns on me that I am breathing and my breath could run out. Perhaps I am breathing shallow and there is little breath left in me. I gasp and grab a breath and become conscious of the rhythm. More likely I was deep in thought or deed and so intense that holding my breath was not noticed. Or was I bending and holding my breath? Breathing now has my full attention.

Breathe on me, breath of God,
Fill me with life anew.[6]

After a surgery, the physical therapist told me to keep breathing when I bend over or stretch or exercise. I try to remember, so as to overcome the dangerous feeling of smothering.

Sometimes I feel I am under water and drowning. I went under in Koenig's Sea in Europe, and still feel the fright of that afternoon; that was sixty years ago. I was drowning; Jim saved me.

My breathing seems shallow. It could be phlegm caught, a deception—or the weather, sinus, lungs, bronchitis. All these can do me harm; some are life threatening. Read any death notice; some of these kill. Breathing is harder today than yesterday; it's Friday, too late to call a doctor. But there is always the emergency room. Oh, the wait! The more I watch my breath the worse my breathing. A doctor once assured me that breathing will continue. I need not focus on the process to keep it going. I breathe when asleep or when very busy or occupied.

But this breath is different. I am afraid of breathing; I am afraid of not breathing. My own pattern of breathing is what I fear most. It is for now a worst enemy.

As a religious person, I consider breath important, because breath and energy and spirit and life are synonyms. My breath is the breath from God, of God. Breath means Zoe—life—and that is my granddaughter's name. Why is breath a trouble maker?

Twenty-five years ago the therapist said: "Keep breathing in whatever you're doing." I remember other good sayings that are rooted in me. I have practiced them, over and over; I do again.

I breathe deeply and evenly. In, through the nose, out, through the mouth, over and over, once more. This feels good. There is nothing to worry about. I can go back to what I was doing; I am cured; I am well, but not always. Again, while I pay no heed, anxiety clicks in and I listen to my breathing. Where is it? Why is my breath so quiet, so far away? I inhale quickly to make sure I have enough wind to get me through this new episode.

I exhale confidently; my lungs fill up. I am relieved. Why does it take so many years to learn to breathe right? Sometimes I still fear running out of breath. I am learning to exhale.

O God, this is your breath of life in me. I am afraid to let it go. It is your breath so there is enough. Friends say so; the doctors say so. I know life is your constant gift to me. I have breathed this breath mostly unknowingly for eighty-two years. O Lord, your earth is full of good breath, enough to inhale, enough to exhale. You fill me with life day and night, while aware and when unaware. I know and I forget; I trust and I am afraid. I am like a yo-yo; I leave your hand, I return. I spin like a top; I whirl with joy and I wobble and fall. I am firm and steady. I am weak and weary. People see me brave. I whimper like a prophet caught under water. Woe is me, I am a fearful poet. You know me best. I am afraid, but not afraid to cry: "My Lord and my God." You do not stop knowing me.

— An idea to practice —

Thinking about breathing—or not breathing—can get you into trouble. Just be aware of your breathing, without thinking. Focus your awareness on the rise and fall of your abdomen or the rise and fall of your chest or the feeling of the air moving in and out of your nostrils. Just watch; don't think. Don't try to control your breath; just watch it as it is: rough or even, shallow or deep, fast or slow. Just watch. Watch with gratitude—breath is both life and gift—but don't think; breathe, watch. In this way you will begin to create a space of peace, of calm, of silence within where anxiety's claims upon you lessen. And as you breathe, remember that Jesus "emptied himself." This may be your best practice and it is lifelong. As you breath allow God's breath, presence, Spirit to fill you. This means taking in God with each breath. Remember the hymn: "Breathe on me breath of God, fill me with life anew." Be still. Know God is God. God's presence can fill you from head to foot. Remember the anthem: "God be in my head and in my understanding." Be filled, overflowing with God's life, breath.

- 4 -

Anxiety

Easily Startled

Have no fear, little flock;
Have no fear, little flock,
For the Father has chosen
To give you the kingdom,
Have no fear, little flock.[7]

Sometimes I am easily startled by a single thought, a sudden idea. I become so absorbed by a new thought I am writing or thinking that I startle, frightened, overwhelmed. My body is taken captive by a moment. Opening a can of soup with difficulty, pondering a problem, and I am drained, weakened, as though I have been running and am exhausted; I am fearful.

I can watch a broken tree limb and look so closely that I feel the brokenness, even the pain, and my mind goes to some time when I was in great need. I will not dismiss a bent tree or hail-pounded nature easily. The harm in nature will either startle me or hold me in bondage. I embody the hurt. I will stay with something broken like a friend in need. When finished looking or writing or remembering, I then come up for breath. How quickly I hear life say "Boo!"

A news headline or single sentence on any page can reach out and grab me, hold me, engross me, scare me. I can feel what is not written. A piece of news can cause me to embrace a friend or relative. A printed scenario can take me on an unwanted emotional journey so I am transported to the scene itself. It can put me into a far-flung war zone or trap me in a collapsed bridge in China. I feel the forty hours or ten days a victim is unable to move. I can feel the thirst and hear the cry within fainting silence and watch hope build and then disappear. I pray for dogs to find me and for the touch of a rescuer. I am startled and I am trapped in a few seconds, sometimes quicker.

When I "come to myself," I am often tired, weary, worried, afraid. Often the moment is so traumatic I savor it; it will become a song, a prayer, the theme for a retreat. It is moment I will not easily waste; it is a time I may not face again; but I do. I like surprise; I do not enjoy being startled.

Have no fear, little flock;
Have no fear, little flock,
For the Father has chosen
To give you the kingdom,
Have no fear, little flock.

God, how quickly I startle. A branch breaks, a headline is too
loud, a warning is too sudden, a thought is too strong. Lord,
I am still a lamb, not yet a sheep. I am still learning to know

14

your voice from that of an intruder. I hear my name the way you have called me from the beginning. Sometimes I do not trust my hearing; I trust you but not always myself. I jump like a lamb hearing the howl of an enemy, the snap of a twig, when hid in a valley and unable to see the flock or when the sun sets too soon. I am sometimes too weak, too weary, and do not know my name. I am hid in fear and there is little light around me. Waken a light within me to show me the flock. Sometimes we frighten together and huddle quickly. We are not frantic with a good shepherd in our midst.

My confirmation hymn reads: "Jesus, Still Lead On." That was sixty-six years ago. The hymn is still finding root in me. I cling to the tree. I cling to the flock.

If the way be drear, if the foe be near,
Let no faithless fears o'ertake us,
Let not faith and hope forsake us;
Safely past the foe to our home we go.[8]

— An idea to practice —

Sometimes when we are startled, the ground shifts, and we lose sight of the promises that have sustained us before and can do so again. We get lost in the unexpected or the unimaginable as we play sudden scenarios out in our minds—thoughts and feelings captured by the unforeseen moment. At such times, it helps to return to the source of comfort and strength—the promises and presence of the Good Shepherd. At such times, you might softly pray:

The LORD is my shepherd, I shall not want.
He makes me lie down in green pastures;
 he leads me beside still waters;
 he restores my soul.
He leads me in right paths
 for his name's sake.
Even though I walk through the darkest valley,
 I fear no evil;
 for you are with me;
 your rod and your staff—
 they comfort me (Psalm 23: 1-4).

- 5 -

Anxiety

God

Thomas, lay your finger in my hand and my side.

O God, you are my God, I seek you,
my soul thirsts for you;
my flesh faints for you,
as in a dry and weary land where there is no water.
So I have looked upon you in the sanctuary,
beholding your power and glory.
Because your steadfast love is better than life,
my lips will praise you.
So I will bless you as long as I live;
I will lift up my hands and call on your name.
My soul is satisfied as with a rich feast,
and my mouth praises you with joyful lips
when I think of you on my bed,
and meditate on you in the watches of the night;
for you have been my help,
and in the shadow of your wings I sing for joy
Psalm 63:1-7.

I could have written this psalm by heart when I was ten. It was all so clear; God was not a problem. I knew it the way I felt it on mother's lap.

If mother was anxious, I felt it. Her apron often sheltered me. We shared being anxious; we shared bravery. My father's stories were true and clear, and I believed every word just the way he told it, and the way it was written. He was glad when I said God's words out loud. I knew how to plead, thank, intercede, and praise.

When our family was safe inside the Bible, in prayer, at the kitchen table, I could fight Goliath. Now I am not thinking about my father talking or the word written. I am thinking about my feelings, thoughts, images of God, my trust. What is missing? It is easy to trust when you are a child on the lap of a believing mother or watching father's face when he tells what he believes. They are no longer here, yet I hear them, often too faintly.

Lord, am I alone or lonesome? The dining table was sold in an auction sixty years ago. Perhaps mom's apron is stored in an Omaha closet. The Bible was in German and is a souvenir. Father and mother no longer hold me at the end of the day and tell me the truth. I find their words in print. There is no recording from them. My children are thousands of miles apart. They know of my wants and fears. We have shared our weakness and strength, like in the psalms. We are fearless differently. You know our names and we know places you reveal the truth.

Now there is no lap and no father's voice and face. Years have passed since that time. I have thoughts I did not have then, have heard ideas mother never heard, have read what father may not ever have thought.

Trust is a very big word. Trust is hard without the face of a father or the lap of a believing mom. Not all dads or moms or preachers are the same. As a child I never met an atheist, was never tested by an unbeliever. But now even their thoughts can be my thoughts, and their belief can excite me or tempt me. Eighty years makes a difference. God has more sides than ever; each has a believer. My friends do not agree on one creed. When I was little, we were all of one mind. There were no questions or doubts. If there were differences, we did not mention them. By now I have heard and seen everything. Some say God has many faces. Some are sure of one God, some say there are many. Some are sure science says it all. I believe in all the above.

It is comforting to be in a church pew and go back to child-faith. In my child is the root of my trust. But the root has grown. The branches have lengthened and budding twigs have frozen with late cold so the summer bloom is light. My roots do not always bear good fruit, or enough. The branches are empty, and my soul bears a weak harvest. My heart cries out for help. I am a psalmist; I know by my words: "Lord, I believe; help my unbelief" (Mark 9:24).

Jesus, I need to lay my finger in your side and touch your wounds. I need a lot of proof for a little while. Where is my mother's apron? Where is the kiss and make well? Where is father's sure faith? Where are you, Jesus? "Here I am: in the voice of a son, the smile of a grandchild, a love note on the refrigerator door, Emily who laughs when she sees you at church, the faith of Tom, the hugs of Lisa."

Lord, I believe; help my unbelief.

— An idea to practice —

Anxiety often resides in the collision between certainty and doubt, in the paradox: "I believe; help my unbelief." When such anxiety arises in the strange mix of certainties and doubts, it is best to give it words, voice, expression. Read the ancient Hebrew poets who wrote the Psalms and find words of praise and complaint, trust and doubt that resonate and give voice to the present state of your own soul, mind, heart. And then you might write your own psalm, chanting forth both trust and lamentation, songs and sighs. You hear the words; God hears the words, listening, as God does, with love.

- 6 -

Anxiety

Anticipation

Believers hurried to the grave
The angels met them there
The One they knew who came to save
Was gone; they looked most everywhere.
He told them oft that he would rise
Yet they were not prepared;
So great the fear in this surprise
They left the tomb quite scared.

I remember when little that if I expected something, I would grow silent in anticipation. Why? This waiting was crucial. This was the time to feel the joy and pain of waiting in the same breath. I waited for the moment, the minute the folks returned from a trip; for six in the evening when Winifred would drive in with a candy truck and stay overnight. I anticipated with all my heart. I waited for the event, for the precise moment, not to miss it when it is there. What if they did not return? What if he

21

did not come? I was more silent than still. I still feel this quiet anxiety.

My body and mind still play leapfrog, being sure I will not miss an appointment, or be late. I would rather wait an hour than be five minutes late. I anticipate with bated breath. I do not want someone holding me back. What if the phone rings and I do not hear it? What if Wilfred and the candy truck do not come?

What is the bated breath? I felt it waiting for birthdays and for Christmas Eve to finally come. Waiting was especially painful when I stood at a north window in the country and stared, watching for father's car lights to come down a country hill, turn west and be home, finally, and safe. How quiet I grew during that last mile of rain, fog, mud or snow.

Therefore I tell you, do not worry about your life, what you will eat or what you will drink, or about your body, what you will wear. Is not life more than food, and the body more than clothing? Look at the birds of the air; they neither sow nor reap nor gather into barns, and yet your heavenly Father feeds them. Are you not of more value than they? (Matthew 6:25-26)

Why do Bible verses alone not always help? Why does hope turn so soon to worry? I do not know for how long a time I still stand in my child mind at that north Nebraska window. My emotions trap me. I am absorbed, carried away, transported. When I "come to myself," I am overcome, feeling how much strength has left me. Anxiety has captured me; I am tired. I am not sure Wilfred will come with the candy truck.

Anxiety sucks me into fear and worry. It was so when I was a boy. Sudden turns in the weather, twisters and heavy lightning frightened my mother and also me. Cyclones drove us for safety into the cellar; we huddled in the midst of rural aromas of sauerkraut ripening in huge crocks, apples wrapped in paper for the long winter, and alongside piles of fall potatoes. There in the dark we gathered, knelt, and prayed for safety in the storm. While at play we kept our eyes on the sky to anticipate a storm from a distance, in the next county, and forecast on the radio; once we felt the full wind, breathed the whirling dust and saw debris in the sky as we ran for the cellar door.

My mother would cringe at the clap of sudden thunder. Father soon left and stood on the porch and felt lightning all around. I admired father and clung to mother. I often cling to her anxiety, still, and to father's bravery.

O God, sometimes I stay; sometimes I flee. You know your children. I still flee for my own sake; I hide to live. Often I find this old cellar with earthy aromas inside me; I run and I pray. More and more as I hide, I join millions who are in real trouble. I open my eyes and see I am well after all these years of fear; now it is my time to be with them. You have stayed my course. I give thanks for how you have spared my life. Others around me have fallen; I live. My prayers are the prayers Father once prayed for the family. Now I pray for a new family, beyond kin, beyond this land, in all the world. When I am in my old cellar, somewhere in the world, I find a good refrain that again drives away the foe above the cellar door: "Do not be anxious about tomorrow, for tomorrow will be anxious for itself."

— An idea to practice —

Anxiety that grows out of anticipation of the good happening (What if it doesn't?) or of the bad happening (What if it does?) stunts life, closes it to possibilities beyond the anticipated good or bad. When such anxiety rises within you, focus as much as possible on the possibilities: If not this, then. . . . If this, then. . . . See, feel the largeness of life. Carry a notebook with you: If not this, then. . . . If this, then. . . . Write it all down; expand your boundaries.

Anxiety
Breaking Apart/Racing Thoughts

Just as I am; thy love unknown
has broken ev'ry barrier down;
Now to be thine, yea, thine alone,
O Lamb of God, I come, I come[9]

All my thoughts are breaking apart, separating. I have no more paragraphs or sentences. Words are spinning in all directions like fireworks, but with neither pattern nor beauty. What will I do with this endless stream of thoughts and feelings and words that are breaking apart in me and all around? I am swimming in words; no, I am drowning in words.

My mind has created a black hole to absorb them, and me. It is like a drain in the shower, and thoughts and feelings are disappearing, but not fast enough. There are still more thoughts, more emotions. How can I stop this flood? A million words piling to dim the light in me. A deep, dark hole has formed; a whirlwind of words is hiding the candle. It will burn, later; I know.

Ten days passed, a new song was born; the text says it all: dark hole and a lighted candle.

If all the world came tumbling down
And stars crashed to the ground,
Then hurry, hurry to the One
Who sleeps in hay in Bethlehem
And angels all around.

If devils stood on ev'ry tomb
And filled all hope with gloom,
Then hurry, hurry to the hill
And hear the echo "Yes, I will"
And sea and storm are still.

If all the earth were hill on hill
And ev'ry sound on earth were still
Then hurry, hurry to the place
And hear the angels sing of grace
To all the human race.

O Lord, this is who I am. I know the tomb; I know the tree.
I will not hide from you; I will not let shame keep me from
your pardon. I will not be silent when I am breaking apart.
You know me; this is who I am.

Sometimes I find one word to absorb all rambling words and emotions. It is a very easy word to repeat and image as it absorbs my crumbling world: *Loved. Loved. Loved.*

Just as I am, thou wilt receive,
Wilt welcome, pardon, cleanse, relieve;
Because thy promise I believe,
O Lamb of God, I come, I come.[10]

St. Paul is right; we are to keep on telling the story of salvation. Not only ponder it, but tell it, be bold in witness. It is my turn to testify. Will they believe me if I am breaking apart? When will I be well? How long, O Lord, how long?

Do not be ashamed, then, of the testimony about our Lord or of me his prisoner, but join with me in suffering for the gospel, relying on the power of God, who saved us and called us with a holy calling, not according to our works but according to his own purpose and grace. This grace was given to us in Christ Jesus before the ages began (2 Timothy 1:8-9).

— An idea to practice —

When anxiety sends unconnected thoughts and feelings racing through your mind and soul, slow them down, bring them back to some shape and order through a single word—*loved.* We are all loved, racing thoughts, tumultuous feelings, and all—*loved, cherished, delighted in.* As you breathe in, repeat this sacred word—*loved.* As you breathe out—*loved.* Breathing in and breathing out—*loved;* breath slowing, thoughts slowing, emotions slowing—*loved.* "Just as I am. . . ."

- 8 -

Anxiety

Need to Talk to Someone

How I loved the setting sunlight
When a day goes fast asleep
And a candlelight stayed burning
When we all lay down to sleep.
I was little and a child
And I hear my family breathe.
Time has moved, I do not hear them;
All is quiet. Did they leave?

I need to talk to someone. It happens a lot. I am overwhelmed with this feeling. Not just anyone but someone who will know what I mean, how I feel, what I am asking. It can be John on the phone, but I have already called him twice this week. It can be Anne, but she is seldom home. It is too late to call the others, like in New York or Florida. I could email, but I need to hear a voice.

What will they say? Last week several said: "Call any time." Did they really mean it? It's after two a.m. and they are asleep. They mean well; can I make it until morning? I have before.

If Lois were here, I could make it. I would reach over and tell her how I feel. She'd ask me to remember what helped the last time, and the hundreds before that. I remember exercises that helped: standing at the side of the bed and stretching, breathing deeply and exhaling slowly, bending and letting my arms hang to the floor. What I want now is a voice; all I need is a good question, an assuring touch.

Now I am alone. There is no voice, no touch, no right question.

Next time I will call someone, or go there, or ask them to come. Not this time. They may not understand this feeling I have. They are not my counselor. I sometimes see them in church and I hardly know them. They volunteered when I mentioned something to them. They may ask me questions I do not want to talk about. After I have explained how I feel, I may be sorry I bothered them. My problem may seem trivial. What if my need suddenly goes away? I can make it through alone, this time; I have before.

God, I have fifty numbers in my phone book, and I am alone. My family's names are all in my cell phone, and I am alone. Thousands know me and would do anything to comfort me, and I am alone. You promise to be with me always, I know where to find this written in the Bible, and I am alone. There are more than two thousand in my parish, and I am alone. There is only a wall between neighbors on either side and below, and I am alone. Once I chose the name of someone

who lives in another country. I gave thanks for everything I
could think you did in this person's life. After thirty minutes,
I was not alone.

For fifty years we sang, often at the living room piano. A hymn sings best when sung with another. We visited more than twenty countries together, saw so much, met so many, then so much to talk about at home. I borrow these times in the night; they keep me company when I choose to be by myself. The only breath I hear is my own; my voice is still. Perhaps the wind out the window will moan; that will help.

Maybe that is why he often phoned at two a.m. He was alone, famous, and alone. I was often with him. One can be famous and cry, be too tired, too still, too depressed. It is why he said he loved Martin Luther. Martin knew the highs and the lows. So he found company with a fifteenth-century minister. Saints and martyrs can help!

O Master, let me walk with you
In lowly paths of service true;
Tell me your secret;
Help me bear the strain of toil
The fret of care.

Teach me your patience;
Share with me
A closer, dearer company.
In work that keeps faith sweet and strong,
In trust that triumphs over wrong.[11]

Every day my children and I are connected. Email, phone! How did my mother and father feel when for years they walked to the country mail box and there was no letter from me? They never said they wanted to talk with me. How did I not know? Now I know.

— An idea to practice —

Anxiety often grows from the soil of grief and loneliness, a prickly shrub that needs trimming back, always. A good way to go about pruning one's spreading sorrow and isolation is to go about blessing others. When loneliness stabs like a sharp thorn and grief spreads its tendrils around your soul, go through every name in your address book, cell phone directory, email contact list; let each one live for a moment in memory and inner vision, and then bless them all one by one with this short prayer:

In the grace and love of God
May you be filled with loving kindness.
May you be well.
May you be peaceful and at ease.
May you be happy.[12]

- 9 -

Anxiety
Excessive Worry

Once there was a child who worried that a seed
she planted might not grow.
Every day she dug it up to look. It did not grow.
She married a farmer and learned to trust.

I trust. I believe. Yet I will stare for hours to make sure it will happen. I will not dig up a seed, but I will make a thought too heavy to move. In a minute I have built a fence into a cement wall.

I can make a mountain out of a molehill. My mindscape can grow too jagged and steep. Suddenly I see old hills and rock slides, and my body feels the rumble of a quake. Little feelings and thoughts grow excessive, and my mind is once again riding a rough road. Why again, and again? I see a mountain expand before my eyes. It is like watching a storm on the horizon come toward my house to threaten all of us. I alone see it and cannot keep it to myself. Like a balloon, the thought must burst. Then it passes. How? Why?

All my early life I watched farmers worry. I lived among them and watched for their worry. There was no irrigation or crop insurance. This was the end of the Depression and the years following. I worried when hail was forecast or when the Long Branch Creek flooded corn and wheat. What I remember most is listening to them on Sunday mornings when they met at church. Old men laughed louder than all, and Mrs. Spilker sang better than ever. In fact, all the farmers sang. I never noticed one quit singing. In these times, I often let a tiny worry get too big.

I do read psalms that comfort; yet I am on this rough road, waiting in the path of a storm, confronting a mountain. I have prayed as have others; yet I am on the rough climb to heights I do not choose and steeps I cannot scale. I hoped this path was past and here it is again. A tiny word has turned into worry.

I have sketched pictures of this journey and written songs so others can avoid the most bumpy path; sometimes a dip turns into a pothole for me. Worry does not offer an easy ride. How did the hill get so high?

So where is *my* help? I have become a guide for many who travel worrisome roads. Is that a gain? Some sing my songs, read my hopeful words, and quit the worry, while I am still on that unhappy way. Where is *my* help?

If lilies of the valley bloom
And are not worry bound
But stand quite tall with open bloom
And roots dug in the ground
Then I do hope what I do sow

Will turn my heart to trust
That when the seed will break to grow
Rain, sun will waken dust.

Friends have brought my own prayers and hymns to my bed for me to read, for my comfort. But I cannot read or sing them now. These words helped me thirty years ago or later, but not now. I do not sing them, because they do not fit me now. Not tonight, maybe tomorrow, but not now. There are other words to help now—or a person or a touch.

I will not waste this worry time. What will it birth? Am I being molded on a potter's wheel? God is the potter; am I the clay?

When I worry, God, I will blow up fifty balloons for fifty wor-
ries until they pop and I will laugh. Will this help? I will find
a circus and choose a ride I fear, and cheer. Will this help? I
will ride a Ferris wheel and sing all the while. Will this help?
I will record my worries for a day and show them to someone
I trust. Will this help? I will admit this is who I am. Will this
help? I will stay still on the potter's wheel. Will this help?

— An idea to practice —

Excessive worries, little worries that mushroom into a mountain of worries, usually don't seem excessive at the time. They sneak up on you and whisper or shout "Boo!" And then it seems too much and too late. Doing things that whisper or shout back "No!" can help make little worries small again. Plant a flower, ride a roller coaster, sing, whistle, walk around with a half smile on your face, laugh for no reason, hug someone, pray, stay on the potter's wheel, wonder what good thing God is making out of you now. Learn or study a new skill—painting, poetry, reading, music, woodwork, knitting—to break your routine and waken new interests. Practicing such skills can absorb anxious times.

10

Anxiety

Closed In

We were children in our home
One painting was a prize
Jesus knocking on the door
The door did open from inside
How we loved this great surprise!

Who locked my door? Why do I feel the windows are shut and locked? I locked them. They lock from the inside. I locked them, but why? I like open windows. Why are they locked this weekend, this night, again?

I crave company. I know I need people and outside and meeting friends; have I locked them out? Why am I locking myself in? Or am I locking the world out? Is it the same?

I pick up the phone to call, then lay it down. I am tired and they will ask "Are you all right?" What do I say? I have highs and lows; they know that. That will not satisfy them. They will want to know more; so do I. Why am I locked in?

Was it something somebody said; am I protecting myself? Is it something I was asked to do and wish not to? Am I preserving my health, my energy, my reputation? This does not feel healthy. What if I went out and did my work poorly? They do not expect me to do poorly in Dallas and Seattle next month. But that is a month away. Am I trying to hide, shutting the door, locking windows?

Listen! I am standing at the door, knocking; if you hear my voice and open the door, I will come in to you and eat with you, and you with me (Revelation 3:20).

Is this my monastic side? Is this part of being a mystic? I need time to reflect, and ponder, and pray. This place is like a desert place, an island, a quiet beach. No, it is more like a prison.

This is more than contemplative and quiet. Why the locked doors and windows? Why the shades drawn? This place is not like an island. How did I build this prison? Why are the shades shut? Will anxiety lock doors?

Knock, knock.
Who's there?
Jesus.
Jesus who?
I thought you knew.

I sat alone at a north window. Lois was sewing and the machine was a friendly sound, when I listened. She hummed as usual. My eyes were closed. Again I had found my own little room. I was sad, alone, rocking. The doors were shut; I sat by a large window.

Peck, peck.
Who's there?
Sparrow.
Sparrow who?
I thought you knew. Chirp, chirp.

O God. I know when you hum. I know when you chirp. I know
when you stay and will not go away. I know when you sing
and I do not hear. I know. You know my secret thoughts, which
I cannot fully understand but which are all known to you.

There is a room in us, locked. Only we have the key. And
also, there is a room we are locked in. And we have the key. For
me it is the same key. I hold the key but too often cannot find the
keyhole. If it is too dark to find the keyhole, I wait for dawn. I
can always count on the rising sun.

Once there was a boy they said was bad. So he grew up bad,
very bad. He was so bad they sent him to his own room; he
had to stay in this room for fifty-five years. He had always
liked his family cabin and went there alone for weeks at a
time, but never for fifty-five years. The room locked only
from the inside. After fifty-five years he could unlock himself.
It was an experiment of a new kind of prison. The warden is
named Jesus.

– *An idea to practice* –

Anxiety certainly can draw the shades and lock the doors and
windows that keep the world out and keep us out of the world.

We become prisoners in a prison of our own making. But Paul said: "For freedom Christ has set us free." And Peter said, "there is no other name under heaven given among mortals by which we must be saved." From the beginning, the name of Jesus has been a prayer expressing faith and trust and love and asking for mercy, peace, forgiveness—the freedom that comes from Christ. As soon as you notice anxiety closing the doors and drawing the shades, begin to repeat the name of Jesus in rhythm with your breathing—a prayer to the One "in whom we live and move and have our being."

11

Anxiety

Tiredness

O Joy, that seekest me through pain,
I cannot close my heart to thee.
I trace the rainbow through the rain
And feel the promise is not vain
That morn shall tearless be.[13]

It's only noon. Tired again; tired yesterday. Will it be the same tomorrow? Sitting at the computer, reading news, and suddenly asleep.

Stress. That's what my friends say. The doctor gave it a name I did not memorize; it is the same. We were talking about anxiety and she said a name, Greek or Latin. She knew. I do not feel pain, like a broken bone; I am tired. A broken spirit.

It's not a disease, like heart failure or lung cancer. Surely it can be cured. I know some things that work, at least for a while, enough to get me going. Then it happens again, so tired.

I put my head on the table and soon disappear. It is as though I sink into a deep hammock and do not want to move, cannot move. Sometimes I yawn and yawn; the breathing wakes me, a little. But I remember the quiet feeling in the hammock and have to keep moving before I give in. I will get through the day. I always do. There is no pain. I will get my thoughts on something else, what else? Can thoughts make me tired?

My nights are short; it has always been so. I can read and write for hours without moving. Now every move is work. I am awake; I stretch. What makes me tired? Stress, they say; you are stressed. Meeting deadlines; but deadlines usually spur me on. Goals draw me, energize me, waken me. How can a deadline make me tired?

If water turns to sweetest wine
And people dance and sing,
Will tired turn to joyous peace
And back to rest again?
If caterpillar turns cocoon,
Then sleep, and butterfly,
Then I asleep in a cocoon
Will wake and break and fly.

I love the sky. I wait for sunsets, stare into them, and rise early for the sunrise. Not now. Now it is not the same. I wake, knowing the color and brightness are around me. Not now. I keep my eyes closed for one more minute of sleep. I do not sleep and I am missing the sun. Alas, I do not care. Not now.

O God, you rested. There is a rest you give creation to make
it whole. Every part of me belongs to every part of me. There
is balance, precise balance. There is wholeness, holiness. It is
a peace that passes understanding. I know that peace. Not

now, but I know it. When it is not in me, I know the peace will come again. You come when the sun shines and I sleep. You come when I stay hid and the doors are shut. You come. I am only tired; I will listen for your words: "Peace I give unto you." Is there a rest, a peace deeper than sleep? Is there a light better than dark?

Awake my heart with gladness,
See what today is done;
Now, after gloom and sadness,
Comes forth the glorious sun.
My Savior there was laid
Where our bed must be made
When to the realms of light
Our spirit wings its flight.[14]

— An idea to practice —

Anxiety can be exhausting, sapping energy, causing the eyelids to droop, moving the mind into the gathering darkness of sleep. Jesus said: "Come to me, all you that are weary and are carrying heavy burdens, and I will give you rest. Take my yoke upon you, and learn from me; for I am gentle and humble in heart, and you will find rest for your souls" (Matthew 11:28-29). A yoke connects or joins together; two oxen or other draft animals are joined with a yoke, making the power of the one available to the other. Imagine yourself "yoked" to Jesus, his power and energy available to you—and then go for a walk, a mile or two or three. And as you walk, don't think about anything—just observe the beauty and wonder of the world.

- 12 -

Anxiety
Depression

My God, my God, why have you forsaken me?
Why are you so far from helping me, from the words of my groaning?
O my God, I cry by day, but you do not answer;
and by night, but find no rest
Psalm 22:1-2.

This was not the first time I was depressed. But it was the first time the nurses and doctor saw my spirit so low. They looked at me to study me and they knew what to ask. I have asked myself the same questions often, which I know by heart. They were not laughing. A young technician came in to draw blood. She was smiling, and humming. I offered her one hundred dollars for her joy. She said she'd give me half of it so I would not have to pay. She took my blood and some of my sadness.

A mood specialist stood by the door and studied me. I could feel her presence and concern. The staff kept asking me about my depression.

Then came some pills, new to me. They made me sleepy, and I knew this was not the solution. It was an experiment. The sadness was my high mountain to climb. I knew some day I would scale this high wall before me. Now I was in a valley. Deeper still, I was in a hole, a deep hole. At the very bottom I knew there was a candle; it was always so. But the candle was not yet lit. I kept saying to visitors, that I would light the candle; sometime. And the candle would give me a new song. It did, but not then. There was no tune in me. Only the quiet, deep moaning of sadness.

A chaplain tested my faith. The questions were not helpful. Another chaplain hugged me. I still feel the touch. I was sure the candle would light; then I would find a new song. The candle did light.

Now you know. Why am I telling you?

My dear clergy friend Don has shared how he lives through depression. He writes: "The St. Barnabas Spiritual Director gave me an assignment one weekend: to write my own lament. What a lament!

> God!
> I would ask Why?! But it's an old question—you can handle so well and I want to ask or say or cry out something that will get your attention and get under your skin.
>
> It goes on and on, this depression. It is so sly and capricious—putting on masks, playing different roles. But always the same result—I despair and have little energy left to fight. I cry out to you. I wait upon you. I

look up to the hills. I come unto you heavy laden. And still it remains. Is it any wonder that I doubt your existence—and you are not even troubled about that.

I hope that in meditation I will be able to open up in the right way if that's what I need to do to realize your loving presence—but the voice that speaks most loudly and clearly is the darkness.

I think at times that I am one continual cry of pain and helplessness—longing for your help. But still it does not come (as I can sense it). You must hear me— you must care—you must want life for me. But nevertheless I find myself left alone and do not sense your presence.

(Then I took a turn that was a gift to me)

In spite of you I will believe and trust that you love, accept, and care for me—and that in your time you will do what needs to be done. I will *hold you to your own words*—and out of even death will expect life. I will do all I can if need be to haunt you with your own promises, plans, and dreams for me. I will not give up on you—ever! To my last dying breath I will wait upon you to deliver the goods, which you yourself have promised. Either I will show you off to be the fraud that you are or will joyfully claim and celebrate the inheritance of one of your children. But, you've got me! For I trust in you, hope in you, believe in you! Help my unbelief![15]

Don trusts and hopes and believes in God. And he needs the Psalms; so do I.

Save me, O God,
for the waters have come up to my neck.
I sink in deep mire,
where there is no foothold;
I have come into deep waters,
and the flood sweeps over me.
I am weary with my crying;
my throat is parched.
My eyes grow dim
with waiting for my God (Psalm 69:1-3).

— *An idea to practice* —

Read through the Psalms; notice all the feelings you feel, the highs and the lows. Notice especially the lows, the complaints, the confusion, the hopelessness and despair, the anger—all voiced to God by these ancient people of faith, apparently with the confidence that God can take it. When the coiling miasma of depression settles over you, take up pen and paper (or keyboard) and write your own lament, give voice to what is real with you; God can take it.

13

Anxiety

Roller Coaster

Once upon a time a little girl loved riding roller coasters.
When summer came, she could ride one for hours at the county fair.
She is older now and has no time for county fairs.
But she is on a roller coaster and wants off.
It is there wherever she goes.
Her son would like to help her get off,
but he is too little to stop the wheel.
She would take him with her,
but it is not the kind of roller coaster she remembers
from the county fair.

Time goes by so fast; there is no time for rest. Day after day, big and little things are on a roller coaster; many seem the same, touching, overlapping, blurred. Where is the space between? Where are the times and places to rest?

Sometimes I am bored. Not with nothing to do, but with the rush, the same going, going, going.

The days have lost their rhythm and blend into sameness. Sameness is tiring. I need rest, even a day of rest, a minute. I need resting times along the way, to reflect, to see where I am, what is around me; to see a blossom, one bloom, to bend over a bush to see leaves up close, to know the aroma. How did this roller coaster happen, and why? I do not see the stars, the night sky, the sunset. I rush into the day and on into the night. Sometimes it is the same, hurry, hurry, deadline, deadline. What is driving me so?

> *O God, it seems I go, go, go, and I give, give, give. There is no time to receive. I am too busy, too tired to receive. There is not time to be served, cared for, helped, not time to ask. It is not a vacation I need, but times of rest, sabbath rest. Tiny times of sabbath time. God, on the seventh day you took a rest. Each day of creation you blessed what was done. When is there time for me to bless each day what I do, and you do? I am losing the rhythm of life. It is all one straight, fast line. One straight line of heart rhythm means death. Am I dying? The seasons in each day are blurred. The weeks have lost their rhythm. In the swift doing of things I am often bored. The speed has blurred life into sameness.*

What did Jesus say when he went off alone to pray? What do monks think and say and do to find rest and sabbath in their solitude? What do people pray on battlefields and in strafed homes and bombed villages? How do people who show strength find rest and peace in the midst of chaos and hell? How are children not numbed by the same horrors week after week? What do children imagine and play, how do they rest while I ride this roller coaster?

Who will be my mentor?

Come to me, all you that are weary and are carrying heavy burdens, and I will give you rest (Matthew 11: 28).

– An idea to practice –

Anxiety can keep you too busy, running too fast. It is hard to get off the roller coaster when you are always in the place where the roller coaster runs. It is hard to smell the roses when you tear by the roses so fast, always so fast. Henry David Thoreau, the hermit of Walden Pond, wrote that he went to the woods because he wanted "to live deliberately." How delicious that sounds—to live deliberately, not pushed and pulled in a thousand different directions at once by the always running riptides of anxiety. Perhaps we could learn from Thoreau and go to the woods every now and then, away from the places where the roller coaster runs. Find a hermitage or retreat center where you can go for sabbath rest for a weekend or a week; walk in the woods, smell the world, feel the rhythms of the Lord of the Dance, the One in whom there is real rest.

14

Anxiety

Now

There comes a twister!
We saw them coming across Nebraska fields
and chose the little ones to stand in,
in the very center, and to feel the calm.
The dust on us was worth the moment.
We stood in a moment of awe.
The twister kept moving, faster than we could run.
That moment, that Now was a very great experience.

I am surrounded by now, overwhelmed with this hour, minute, moment. The past is in me, rushing through my mind. Not in an order of events, more like a collage. Fifty years ago and twenty and forty and two all at the same time. They are all inside this moment. Names loom large of Sister Marie Louise, Bishop Sheen, Buchenwald, my country school mates, Joe Louis, President Roosevelt, Aunt Minnie in Pittsburgh, Gertrude in Holden Village, Thomas from Berlin. All these flash into my mind; it is a huge blur of thoughts, pictures, events and feelings. My now is overflowing. There is no more room and still the past keeps filling my thoughts.

The future does the same. What will happen, could happen, comes racing into me. How will it be with my grandchildren in ten years, in America in fifty years, the environment? All these are part of now, uninvited, loud. How can I live in the present, this moment, when I am so overwhelmed? Where are the doors to guard this moment? I want to be restful, quiet, gentle enough to enjoy. I do not like this flood.

I pray, and no sentence gets finished. My petitions tumble over each other; there is no logic. It is the way I scribbled as a child when I did not know what to draw. The lines and circles filled the paper. My thoughts make my mind dark, one enormous scribble. All I want is a simple picture of today.

Sixty years ago I learned to play one song on the piano.

Now is the hour, when we shall say goodbye;
Soon you'll be sailing far across the sea.
While you're away, oh please remember me;
When you return, you'll find me waiting here.[16]

Now I am not on a journey. I am trapped inside now. I am looking in all directions without moving. The more my mind turns to see what is entering me, and wakening in me, the more quiet my body grows. I sit still and stare. How do I stop the flow, the flood, the mental cyclone, the emotional twister?

Then the Lord answered Job out of the whirlwind: "Gird your loins like a man; I will question you, and you declare to me. Will you even put me in the wrong? Will you condemn me that you may be justified? Have you an arm like God, and can thunder with a voice like his? Deck yourself with majesty and dignity; clothe yourself with glory and splendor" (Job 40: 6-10).

I scream. I recall the painting "The Scream" by Edvard Munch and feel someone else knows this whirlwind. I hear the silent scream from the mouth on the canvass and receive some comfort.

God, sometimes I scream
As though it is your fault
And you do not leave me or scold me
Nor did my mother
And then I helped her with the dishes
I still feel the warm soapy water.

Incline your ear, O LORD, and answer me,
for I am poor and needy.
Preserve my life, for I am devoted to you;
save your servant who trusts in you.
You are my God;
be gracious to me, O Lord,
for to you do I cry all day long.
Gladden the soul of your servant,
for to you, O Lord, I lift up my soul.
For you, O Lord, are good and forgiving,
abounding in steadfast love to all who call on you
(Psalm 86:1-5).

— An idea to practice —

When your now is filled with past and future, your now is an illusion, because the past was not how we remember it and the future, when it gets here, will not be as we imagined it. What's real is not what happened or what will happen, but what is happening right now. Pick up an orange; roll it between the palms of your hands, feel its roundness. Peel it, slowly, very slowly; feel the texture of the orange skin, smell the orange scent as it rises from the split skin to your nose, feel the cool juice run from your fingers to the palm of your hand and up your sleeve. Arrange the peels carefully on the countertop, one piece on top of another, a small tower of fragrant orange peels. Tear off a piece of the now peeled orange and place it on your tongue; chew it slowly, thirty times before swallowing, taste it. Repeat with another piece and another until the orange is gone. You have just spent several minutes in the present moment, in now without past or future crowding in.

Anxiety

Weather

We plow the fields and scatter
The good seed on the land,
But it is fed and watered
By God's almighty hand.
He sends the snow in winter,
The warmth to swell the grain,
The breezes and the sunshine,
And soft refreshing rain.[17]

In our country church schoolhouse we sang this song—*Wir Pfluegen und Wir Streuen (We Plow the Fields and Scatter)*—in two languages, over and over through the years. There was no weatherman on WCCO, Omaha; there was God.

Is it you God, or the weatherman? Or both?

I was raised to believe God did the weather. Psalm 104 was too long for me then, but this is what we believed in our home and world.

> *Bless the LORD, O my soul.*
> *O LORD my God, you are very great.*
> *You are clothed with honor and majesty,*
> *wrapped in light as with a garment.*
> *You stretch out the heavens like a tent,*
> *you set the beams of your chambers on the waters,*
> *you make the clouds your chariot,*
> *you ride on the wings of the wind,*
> *you make the winds your messengers,*
> *fire and flame your ministers.*
> *You set the earth on its foundations,*
> *so that it shall never be shaken (Psalms 104:1-5).*

Weather was a worry when I was little. Farmers had neither irrigation nor crop insurance. For months during worship, father pled in prayer for right weather. Work and bread and butter depended on good weather. I watched the faces of farm families while father prayed. They seemed hopeful, trusting, less anxious than I.

I was sad when insects stripped the cornstalks and ate heads of farmers' grain. I worried that rust would spoil a good wheat crop. I felt God sent a plague when hail crushed good grain to the ground. Though far from Egypt, I argued with God about weather and justice. God was the only weatherman I knew.

We watched the sky and wind and clouds for any sign of the weather we needed, prayed for, and expected. More and more I expected the good weather father prayed for. Even though he prayed "Your will be done," I knew what my will was.

We did not know what the weather reports now tell in detail. We did not understand weather patterns and systems and fronts. Weather was about God and prayer and how we lived our lives. Bad weather could make me feel like a bad person. A farmer spared of hail was special and blessed. If our garden was destroyed, there was a lesson to be learned, but I did not know what that meant.

So I learned to feel some responsibility and control in matters of weather. Weather was a spiritual affair and a matter of prayer. I often find myself drawn between God and the weatherman in matters of storms, floods, tornadoes, and crop failure.

Weather can create anxiety. I can easily feel these concerns: What if it rains during the parade? What if there's a blizzard on Christmas Eve? What if our picnic is rained out? What if it's too hot for the walk? What if it hails on the crops? What if the levees break?

Once there was a weatherman who was religious. He studied weather, and he believed in God. He always prayed while preparing his forecasting. He believed that after he reported to the people, then it was God's turn. He prayed that God would move the people to be just and grateful after a good rain, a storm, a flood, a tornado, or a plague of rust. He knew what to say on the news about climate and atmosphere but he could not control the hearts of the listeners after a gentle shower or a ravaging storm. There was plenty for God to do.

God was my father's weatherman.

It was often true
Mother earth was parched and dry
As child I bent to hear her cry
And when rain came, father lifted high his hat
And like in church he bowed his head
I did not hear just what he said.
So now I too would do just that
If rain came just right and if I wore a hat.

I listen to the weatherman; I thank the Lord.

All good gifts around us
Are sent from heav'n above.
Then thank the Lord, oh, thank the Lord
For all his love.[18]

— An idea to practice —

Weather can indeed be a source of anxiety, and like most sources of anxiety, it is completely out of our control. Weather can bring harm or good. It can both delight and torment—sometimes both at the same time. The farmers' delight at the drenching, drought-busting rain is the partygoers' torment when the long-planned picnic is ruined. Weather can also be violent; it can kill—*the price we pay* for living in a scientifically explainable universe. And it can bring with it the most exquisite beauty, *the price we are paid* for living in a scientifically explainable universe. When a sudden cloud rains on your parade, what to do except to try "singing in the rain." "Then thank the Lord, oh, thank the Lord for all his love," a love that can be known in all kinds of weather.

- 16 -

Anxiety

Failure

"Carl, do they know their names?"
"No, I know their names. They know my voice."
"How do they come home?"
"I call and they come running."

Carl was eighty-five; he had one hundred two sheep. Carl was once a custodian.

"For nothing will be impossible with God." Then Mary said, "Here am I, the servant of the Lord; let it be with me according to your word." Then the angel departed from her (Luke 1:37-38).

Mary, a teenage Judean girl said to Gabriel, "So be it." She was humble; she did not fear failure.

Carl was a custodian; he understood calling. Mary was a young Judean girl; she understood calling. I was raised on the word calling, *Berufung*. Why this feeling of failure?

All life is to be sacred. I was raised not to fail. I could come in second or third, but I would not fail. Even last place was not to be understood as failure. Sights were high; growing up was a test. So I have often won in life, and failed. If I see myself coming in last, I make plans to improve, but not always.

I skipped grades in country school and was out of college at age eighteen. I gained, I lost.

We were taught to be thorough: pick every potato bug in the field, pick every mulberry, and get every spelling word right. Our homework was drilled and we knew how to cook, fry, peel, iron, clean. I plowed and ran tractors and combines at an early age, and I drove when twelve. We hired out young to milk, shock grain, thresh and hay. We were expected to do our best, and even excel. We were not taught to fail. All life is to be sacred. Do your best, and better.

Fear of failure creeps into my mind. I feel this fear in my spirit; I can feel torn, bursting, exhausted, depressed. I have learned to shout to God by name. "My God! Jesus Christ!" How often I have made the sign of the cross before me! I cast out fear with the name of God whose voice I know. Oh yes, I know the name and I say the name aloud. I may come in last but I will not fail. I will learn as I stumble; I will grow as I fall and am helped up. And yet I holler, "Help!" And I sometimes lose my voice.

I am a called person. I do not want to be driven or pushed or shoved or neglected. I want to be called, expected to do well, chosen. I want to be perfect. Seventy-five years ago I memorized: "Be perfect, therefore, even as your heavenly Father is perfect" (Matthew 5:48). I keep learning what this means to me. I have more and more possibility, potential. I need not fail. God keeps encouraging me, drawing me out, growing me.

I feel failure when pushed and shoved. I feel success when called. I do not like a voice shouting, "Thou shalt! You should!" I like the still small voice whispering, "You are able. I want you." I answer, "Here I am, Lord, send me."

I see a font, I hear calling. I see a river, I hear a voice: "Beloved." I once dared ask a group, "Who am I to you? Who do you say that I am?" They answered, "Beloved." For years when an anxious day haunted me with the words: "Who are you?" I repeated as mantra, "Beloved. Beloved. Beloved."

Then one of the seraphs flew to me, holding a live coal that had been taken from the altar with a pair of tongs. The seraph touched my mouth with it and said: "Now that this has touched your lips, your guilt has departed and your sin is blotted out." Then I heard the voice of the Lord saying, "Whom shall I send, and who will go for us?" And I said, "Here am I; send me!" (Isaiah 6:6-8).

When I hear my name being called, I come running.

I heard the voice of Jesus say,
"I am this dark world's light;
Look unto me, your morn shall rise,
And all your day be bright."
I looked to Jesus, and I found
In him my star, my sun;
And in that light of life I'll walk
Till trav'ling days are done.[19]

– An idea to practice –

Nothing learned from—even coming in last—can be called a failure. Learning, growing, maturing, getting better is what life is all about. The true meaning of success has nothing to do with getting power, position, prestige, possessions, privilege; it has everything to do with becoming more of who you are. When you feel like a failure, take pen and paper and write down all the things you learned from the experience; write down what you are going to do differently because of the experience; write down how the experience is a part of—and strengthens—your calling from God.

- 17 -

Anxiety

Age

When I was twelve, Mrs. Hertlein must have been forty.
That seemed old at the time.
Persons had to be that old to be more God-like, which she was.
She was beautiful, with one leg shorter than the other. She limped.
What I remember most is that she limped
and smiled at the same time.
I hardly noticed the limp.
The way she smiled almost turned her walk into a swaying dance.
Dancing was not something we were allowed to do,
but watching Mrs. Hertlein seemed like a dance to me.
In her I saw the face of God, the dancing God.
I see it clearly now.
I see that joyful face of God in the song,
"Joyful, joyful, we adore thee."
Mrs. Hertlein's portrait is in a special gallery within me.

When singing a hymn in worship, I always check the date of birth and death of composer and lyricist. I want to know their age, when they lived, and their life and age connection to myself. All ages matter to me. It is true of those around me; all ages are now within me.

> *Guided by the Spirit, Simeon came into the temple; and when the parents brought in the child Jesus, to do for him what was customary under the law, Simeon took him in his arms and praised God, saying,*
>
> *"Master, now you are dismissing your servant in peace,*
>   *according to your word;*
>   *for my eyes have seen your salvation,*
>   *which you have prepared in the presence of all*
>   *peoples,*
>   *a light for revelation to the Gentiles*
>   *and for glory to your people Israel"* (Luke 2:27-32).

Aging has been a lifelong interest. Perhaps because of my brother's traumatic and sudden death when I was nine. I have not been anxious about aging—that is turning thirty or fifty or eighty. What has made me anxious is running out of years. From childhood I did not think my life would be long. I felt it would be full and fulfilling, but not lengthy. It has been both. I was ready to go, but not at all willing.

So, there have been more times than I can count when I feared aging in some way. I feared an illness that would shorten my years or end my years with pain and depression. I have feared sadness as a final illness. It is hard for me to come to terms with unfinished business.

O Lord, will my legacy be tears? What will mark my grave stone? What will I leave that shall not die? How long will the songs live, and who will remember my thoughts? Who will say my name and who will remember my years? Who will know what is stored in tubs in my garage that I will not have time to open? Who will know the archives in my mind? Will it be you? You, O Lord?

As a child I borrowed illness in farm families as though I was the next to have polio, tuberculosis, a stroke, or any disease painful or fatal. Aging then had less to do with growing older and more about suffering with aging. As years pass, I am amazed at how I have lived long and full. Nevertheless, the anxiety that goes with aging can frighten and depress me. My spirit is willing and my flesh is weak.

Health was always greatly on my mind. I had rickets and later wore a body brace. I wanted to play baseball; I had early heart disease. "Please no serious illness." I had cancer surgery. "Strengthen my heart." I had six bypasses, seven stents, and three pacemakers. "Give me a glad spirit." I have had bouts of depression. My brother died when I was nine. I began to draw and to write; I am still writing.

Lord, you have given me years of advocates and support in family, friends, parishes, readers, strangers. Family has sat at my bedside through long night watches, with patience and love, as I more than a few times trembled and feared the dark and tomorrow. Day after day, year after year you have given me life beyond my fears. You have not tired of my whining and sadness; you have given me a dawn I did not expect and grandchildren I did not believe I would see. In the middle of

an anxious time, you have cleansed my spirit. I have lived to
claim your free spirit. You do not tire of my moaning. I am
now gray; you have me feeling younger.

— *An idea to practice* —

Aging can indeed lead to anxiety, because it leads us closer to
the unknown—and raises worries about what the path to the
unknown will be, and will be like. Aging has its downside:
declining health, loneliness as loved ones leave first, perhaps
regrets for things dreamed of but left undone or underdone. But
aging also has its upside: memories, experiences, maturity and
wisdom, perhaps grandchildren, a growing acceptance of the
coming darkness with the trust that in the darkness there is infinite light, there is love. When the inevitability of aging translates
into anxiety, it is good to remember those whose own aging has
already moved them into God's future, good to celebrate their
lives and their returning to the love from which they came. Buy
a journal and begin to write your own story—even if you (and
God) are the only ones who will ever read it. Write down all the
lives that have touched you and all the lives you have touched
in the intricate tapestry of family and friends that is your unique
story, the fruit of your aging.

Anxiety

Self-Image

Please! I do not want to go out of existence!
No, no. Do not erase me.
Cleanse, renew, rebirth, transform, transfigure, recreate me!
Please do not erase me.
I am not an annual.
God, surely I am a perennial!

These have often been my fighting words.

> *But we have this treasure in clay jars, so that it may be*
> *made clear that this extraordinary power belongs to God*
> *and does not come from us. We are afflicted in every way,*
> *but not crushed; perplexed, but not driven to despair.*
> *(2 Corinthians 4:7-8).*

What a relief when I focus on me, Herbert Fredrick Broker-ing, in a new body and a new earth, but not "out of existence."

The I Am stays; Herbert stays. Changes? Yes. New? Yes. Life? Eternal Life? Sure? Yes. How sure? The promise.

Who decides? God! The one who made me and called me and gives me breath of life and mind and soul and health—this God will do it. I trust God to keep me in existence. The God who did it and does it will do it.

God. The God. The God who created me and all that exists. God keeps me and will keep me in existence. How? God knows. Why? Love.

When am I most anxious? When do I worry most? When I pretend to keep myself in existence; when I give Herbert the power and the glory; when I forget a favorite psalm. Psalm 139 quiets me: wherever I go, you are there! Left, right, high, low, out, in, above, below; you are there. In the inner parts: in mother's womb, in semen, in the liver, the heart, the kidney, the mouth, in the cerebellum, in tendons, in DNA, in arteries, in the left ventricle, in the spleen, in the memory—*You are there!*

So we do not lose heart. Even though our outer nature is wasting away, our inner nature is being renewed day by day. For this slight momentary affliction is preparing us for an eternal weight of glory beyond all measure, because we look not at what can be seen but at what cannot be seen; for what can be seen is temporary, but what cannot be seen is eternal (2 Corinthians 4:16-18).

Why does this verse, which I memorized in two languages in 1940, take on new and comforting meaning this Sunday evening while I write to you?

A wise old woman from Mississippi said she was "de lady of de Lawd." She had that kind of connection with God. She knew she would be changed in the twinkling of an eye and not ever be erased. A famous historian and reformer often winked when he prayed. He said, "God is my best friend, a friendship that will not end." He winked again. When I try to save myself I hear Emma and I see Roland and I lose myself. So I find myself.

For more than twenty years I led pilgrimages into many lands. I went as a pilgrim, finding the Way, a minstrel seeking the fountain of youth. I think I was walking my father's journey, an immigrant, I felt, was always homesick. Strangers helped me find Herbert Brokering. Strangers became best friends. So I find myself.

Every people seemed to know a song. Sometimes I need a Messiah or a Good Shepherd or a Mediator or a Savior or a Counselor; sometimes I mostly want a Friend. When pastors gathered in our house in my child days, their talk in three languages about Angels and the Christ's Second Coming and Repentance did not impress me most. What meant most was how these fourteen loved one another. I could have sung "What a friend we have in Jesus." They were Jesus with beards and shaven and bald and cigars and homegrown tobacco stuffed in pipes and Bibles and Greek books wide open. They laughed and prayed and were serious and argued, and knew each other's names. Mostly, they were friends, Jesus-like to me.

No one said anything about going out of existence, now or ever.

In the church where I worship, there is a cross of brass that shines and reflects like a mirror. Sitting near the front and to the side I can see many faces of my church friends reflected, while singing, praying, passing the peace, and smiling. I am better in worship when little Ava sits in the bench ahead of me, and turns to see me. These are the people around me who tell me who I am. They are in me and I am in them. Their joy and stories and hope and fears and faith and pain and voices are in me. I do not do well, in defining myself, by staring straight into a mirror at myself. I do better side-glancing, seeing myself a bit from the side through a host of saints, ten or one thousand in a room in worship. Scattered throughout the room, and between their faces, are martyrs and saints of old and ancestors and unborn. This parade of faithful tell me who I am. When I do not see them I am frightened. Once they needed to be Lutheran or Christian. That is no longer true.

More and more "Who I Am" is a matter of relationship. I am not just me for myself; I know myself when I think and feel and act in relationship. That is true with other persons; they define me. It is ultimately true with God, who defines me in relationship. For years, when more anxious than I can describe, I repeated this phrase with my breathing for hours: "Child of God, Child of God, Child of God."

In Psalm 8 David sings a song about the majesty and position we have with God: "Yet you have made them a little lower than God, and crowned them with glory and honor (v. 5).

Surely this makes me more than a perennial.

— *An idea to practice* —

Who am I? Will I always be, somehow? Do I matter? To God? These are anxiety producing questions. When they rise in your mind, remember that you are now and you are God's. Bless your body, slowly, from feet to head. Do what Psalm 139 does; know that God is present in all parts of yourself. Who am I? Will I always be? Should these questions wend their way into your mind and give birth to anxious thoughts of mortality, counter them with this answer of faith:

> *Do not fear, for I have redeemed you;*
> > *I have called you by name, you are mine.*
> *When you pass through the waters, I will be with you;*
> > *and through the rivers, they shall not overwhelm you;*
> > *when you walk through fire you shall not be burned,*
> > *and the flame shall not consume you.*
> *For I am the LORD your God,*
> > *the Holy One of Israel, your Savior. (Isaiah 43:1a-3a)*

- 19 -

Anxiety

Property

So God created humankind in his image,
in the image of God he created them;
male and female he created them.
God blessed them, and God said to them,
"Be fruitful and multiply, and fill the earth and subdue it;
and have dominion over the fish of the sea and over
the birds of the air
and over every living thing that moves upon the earth"
Genesis 1:27-28.

It was the first time we owned property, that is, a plot of ground
and a house. Monthly payment was a new ritual. We were forced
to be faithful, and were for many years; it is paid for. How wealthy
we were, like queen and king, owning house and grass and hillside and oak and elm. It seemed we were having dominion over
goldfinch and cardinals and owls and orioles and turkeys and

pheasant and sparrows and robins and egrets and night sky and sunrise. This was no time for anxiety; this was time for song.

This is my Father's world;
The birds their carols raise;
The morning light, the lily white
Declare their makers' praise.
This is my Father's world.
He shines in all that's fair.
In the rustling grass I hear him pass;
He speaks to me everywhere.[20]

The song was a favorite and *In the Rustling Grass* became the title of my early book in the 60s.

Oh no! An old question raised its ugly head: Where is the property line? Is her grass on my property? Is my tree on his land? How anxious I grew, not about the monthly payment, but about the property line. We could exchange stories, but not land!

The neighborhood had been a pasture; the houses on the street were new. We all owned new land for the first time. It was October, and red oak splashed on the hillside. What worried me most was the property line. It had been surveyed, but were the markers clear?

On one side a surveyor lived who knew the exact line. I was never sure if a tree I planted was too near his line. When the tree bloomed, I was proud of the west side of my property. When the crab apples fell, I feared they would roll into his yard and be my fault. I did not wish to cut down the tree. I was glad when they picked apples and made jam. I felt forgiven; the forgiveness lasted all winter. Then came spring and I worried—sometimes a lot.

A long hill sloped into my yard. The rain from the properties above ran into my yard, and then into the property below us, even into their driveway. I worried how they felt. Whose water was doing the damage, mine or the neighbors' above? This was my first property. The neighbors above were flooding my yard; I did not know them, we were new. But I was flooding my neighbor's yard. We knew each other. What could I do? Who sent the water? Who created the hillsides?

On the east side, neighbors had planted grass six feet into my yard. Not as a favor; they thought this to be their property line. They planted a hedge on my property and a weeping willow from which years later branches fell onto my house. What worried me most was that our young children would stand on the line between our yard and theirs and holler, "Is this our property?" They did not want to be scolded by a new neighbor for playing outside their yard. I worried; I wanted to move. We stayed. Through the years this worry disappeared. It no longer matters, except it did create a lot of anxious time for twenty years, all about one crab apple tree and a beautiful lilac hedge. The hedge blessed us for fifty years with aroma and a good neighbor. The crab apple tree dropped leaves, but filled many jars of sweet jelly.

Do fences make good neighbors?

How shall we love you, holy, hidden Being
If we love not the world which you have made?
Oh, give us deeper love for better seeing

Your word made flesh, and in the manger laid.
Your kingdom come, O Lord; your will be done.[21]

What miracles were at work on that hillside for half a century? The word made flesh, in the manger laid, and hid in the seasons of trees and lilacs and fruit in every season! A "deeper love for better seeing."

We stayed. We shared property lines. After sleepless nights and anxious times my eyes have seen the kingdom come to the pasture. A stranger will soon "own" the hillside with oak and elm and lilacs.

"How shall we love you, holy, hidden Being"

— An idea to practice —

Property, possessions, things, stuff. The accoutrements of life from which we all too often take our identity and stake our claim to importance; the trappings of life that all too often trap us in anxiety as we fret over how to get them, how to keep them, how to protect them, and wonder who we would be without them. Me, my, mine. It is sometimes good to remember that "things" lose their ability to stir up an anxious mind when we, my, and mine are replaced with us, our, and ours. In the Lord's Prayer, we pray to "our Father," not "my Father;" we ask for "our daily bread," not "my daily bread." Sharing is an antidote to anxiety over belongings. "Our" puts a new perspective on what we used to think of as "mine." Relationships, first; things, second—and always in relationships.

20

Anxiety
Being Late

A little girl wanted a watch, but they were too poor.
She came to know her world by heart.
She memorized sunrise, dusk, midnight, tides, full moon,
slow and fast;
she played piano with a metronome,
knew by heart when it was time for lunch and sleep.
When she was older, she bought a watch,
which she watches as much as she can.
Alas, the watch is now the only way she can tell what time it is.

"I will be on time. In fact, I will be there early! I do not like to be late, so I will not be late. Don't worry; I will not be late!" If I do not say it out loud, I repeat these words clearly to myself for most every appointment, and I have had many.

"And don't anyone make me late!"

Where did this begin? How often this obsession hampered a good beginning, a good trip, a good visit. As a family we would hurry from the house, run to the car to be on time. Often I was at the wheel, engine going, waiting. It was quiet; I was better that way.

Where did this begin? In the country we had chores in the morning; these had to be done so we could walk or ride to the country school on time. If late, we could miss a buggy ride. It might mean walking more than a mile through clay or cold. We would never be late to school or to church or to church school. Others could, and we expected them to come late; we were never late.

I did not mind waiting for a dentist or a doctor or an eye appointment, as was most often the case. They could be forgiven, but not I. I will not be late! A good motto even though mostly filled with fear and anger. What would that say about me, being late?

I liked time. My brother was given a sun dial for his grave stone, which seemed just right to me. He died young; the sun dial continues marking time. I have many clocks in the house, gathered from many places. The sound is like a clock maker's workshop. Quaint. Some do not run; they did run for years. I bought watches from many countries, some twenty years ago, still waiting to be wound. My father's gold pocket watch will run someday. It is sad to be so still.

Years ago, with a box camera, I took time-exposures of night skies. And I wrote about time. I worked the harvest fields. I had no watch; I knew shadows, the sun, dusk and hunger. These kept time for me. Who invented the nine to five time? I spoke against digital time when it first appeared. I missed the fullness of time, the face showing past and present and future.

Then why this anxiety about being late? Time is a precious toy, not a weapon.

Time flows. Time has meter, beats; time dances, plays on tides, rocks. Time unfolds. Signs of time are all around, and in us. Is time meant to be hurried? Are we to make time a threat, a debate? Why would I want to boast: I will never be late?! Is being late bad? The Bible talks about fullness of time but not in anger. Fullness of time is good news!

With all wisdom and insight he has made known to us the mystery of his will, according to his good pleasure that he set forth in Christ, as a plan for the fullness of time, to gather up all things in him, things in heaven and things on earth (Ephesians 1:8-10).

The phrase "fullness of time" intrigues me. God unites all things in a time called fullness of time. How full? Everything at once? Fullness of time: the time when corn is ripe and ready to be husked? The day it's best to cut the barley? This plan of fulfilling time is the plan of Christ. This is gospel time, good news time, a plan with a Christ-like spirit; this time does not yell or glare at a watch while racing the engine. How did time become a law, a threat, a command, a demand? It's time to go, I will not wait! Where does the anger come from?

At eighty-two it is not too late to quit anger, enjoy fullness of time, slow down, ride the tide of time, and make time a best friend. It is not too late to study the skies, learn astronomy, build a clock, give a grandson his first watch. At eighty-two it is the right time to memorize a hymn that sings and celebrates the time and space of God.

God, who stretched the spangled heavens
Infinite in time and place,
Flung the suns in burning radiance
Through the silent fields of space:
We, your children in your likeness,
Share inventive pow'rs with you;
Great Creator, still creating,
Show us what we yet may do.[22]

— *An idea to practice* —

We either live under the tyranny of time or within the mercy of time—it depends on our perspective. Time is either a threat, a sword of Damocles hanging over our head, or grace, a sweet and precious gift of the One who holds everything "infinite in time and space." It all depends on how we look at it. If time's tyranny floods you with anxiety, try taking your watch off for a week, and learn to move to the rhythms that mark the days and nights quite without the need of clock or watch or sundial.

21

Anxiety
Secret

Whoever observes the wind will not sow;
and whoever regards the clouds will not reap.
Just as you do not know how the breath comes to the
bones in the mother's womb,
so you do not know the work of God, who makes everything.
In the morning sow your seed, and at evening do not
let your hands be idle;
for you do not know which will prosper, this or that,
or whether both alike will be good.
Light is sweet, and it is pleasant for the eyes to see the sun.
Ecclesiastes 11:4-7.

I am still learning the work of God. While in darkness, gloom, sorrow, anxiety and depression, God keeps showing light and sweetness. I am in awe!

First I kept the secret to myself. I am not well! While taking medicine for anxiety and heart, I imagined this was minor, like taking aspirin. I traveled far and wide in my work, throughout the states and into many countries. I did not want to be sick or to die. I defied death. Sometimes I felt myself shaking my fist against death. Anxiety was my secret; only my wife and doctor knew. I hardly admitted knowing. I would be all right!

In one decade I was in five ambulances, with sirens shouting. I was getting used to being healed; but I was not healing. I was postponing being well. Driving on Chicago Avenue past the Heart Clinic, I looked the other way. This was not a place I needed. Don't give it a second thought!

After a long while being good at my work and being imaginative and creative, I was told my work was finished. I knew the work was finished and was proud of these years. But they meant something else: "Sorry, the budget cannot afford creativity." I laughed on the outside and cringed within. I studied creativity with the country's best and learned what I was capable of doing. I would freelance my ministry. Three children were enrolling in college and I was promised four hundred dollars for a work in the coming year. Lois prayed; I answered the phone and went to work. Calls took me into towns, cities, colleges, seminaries, Bible camps, military units in the USA and many countries. I had work and often called my doctor from faraway places, asking for help from Berlin, Warsaw, New York, and Canada. I was flown home ill from Berlin, Erlangen, Tokyo, and Saskatoon. I was often frightened, and I lived.

Stress was often discussed with my colleagues. I learned stress exercise that helped me get the strength I was spending in anxious habits. While on the road, I sometimes lay on the floor for hours to be fit for a banquet or workshop. I soon learned how few in the church want to hire someone who might die in their midst. I often wondered why dying was considered a handicap. Could not the death of a guest speaker be a special event?

Lois kept praying, and I answered the phone. There was work to do. She and I could pay the bills and live a good life. The children could continue studying. My ministry on the road and in writing were very productive. I admitted I was racing against fear and death. Through my many surgeries and anxious times, Lois was always beside me, crocheting, reading, praying, humming, caring, and hoping. Hope was near when she was in the room.

The secret is out. I am not always well. I could die en route. I might need an ambulance. This no longer mattered. I was asked to do what I do best. If I am anxious, I still write the hymn, bring stories of faith, pack a surprise, and celebrate with God's people. It is hard to say how much writing this book will depreciate my anxiety. My years have been full and long. I am hopeful this writing will help you, the reader, know a more peaceful life.

For my grave plaque I chose a verse from Philippians: *"May the peace of God which passes all understanding keep your hearts and minds in Christ Jesus."* That is my hope!

My brother fell on water, frozen in December. Death is colder than ice. Since then I have known waters: rivers, fountains, creeks, glaciers, floods, April thaws. I have written many water hymns, filled with awe and hope.

Healing River

O gentle Healing River,
The Jordan hears your Word,
God's Spirit meets the water
And births for us a Lord.
You wash us in a promise,

Beloved is your call;
The one on high in heaven
Is born in cattle stall.

O gentle Healing River,
You grow our desert bloom,
Bring birds into your vineyard,
Your waters wash our gloom.
You flow through silent deserts
For forty days and nights
And when the morning wakens,
You bathe us in God's light.

O gentle Healing River,
You rock us in the womb,
You hold us in a mother
Inside a sacred room.
You birth us to a journey
To sail a sea of grace;
You show your worlds of wonder
To every human race.

O gentle Healing River,
Our brow is never dry,
Once we have touched your water
Our spirits never die.
Pour water, we are thirsty,
Then wash away our tears,
Then give us love and laughter
Inside our earthen years.

O Gentle Healing river,
You wash our blinded eyes
And show us sites for living
Beyond the distant skies.
You are the living water
That flows from Calvary,
Through rivers we now travel
Into eternity.

– An idea to practice –

It is a vicious circle—keeping anxiety a secret creates more anxiety. Do they know? How would they act if they knew? Would they pity me? Look down on me? See me as weak, unable to cope? When anxiety is our secret identity, it is who we are, not just something we are going through. With people you love and who love you, who you care for and who care for you, who you trust and who trust you, why not share the secret? Then it won't be a secret anymore, not who you are, and it will be easier to let others know what you go through from time to time. No shame in that; not at all.

- 22 -

Anxiety

Family

May we all thy loved ones be,
All one holy family,
Loving for the love of thee;
Hear us, holy Jesus.[23]

Once a group of friends went to an open field on a wintry night, lit two candles, placed them in the snow, and drew a circle around them. They stood beyond the circle and sang and prayed. They loved the candles and shared a gentle, brave spirit. They were on the outside and yet felt they were inside the circle. They felt close. Someone threw a snow ball into the circle, then another. One candle went down. Someone hollered: "Stop!" A sad feeling went through the people. It was wartime; many relatives were soldiers. They sang "Silent Night" and quietly left.

I drew a sacred circle around our family. First the circle of father and mother and five siblings in Nebraska. Later the family of Lois and myself and four children. If pain or death came to another family, I hurt and grieved. If it were to visit my family, I did not know how I could bear the grief. In silence, I often practiced a death in my immediate family. I prayed, thanked, pled, and still I felt faint, sweat; my heart pounded or went silent.

What is there about a nuclear family that creates this bond? It was not many years before that we did not know each other. Now we were the tightest community on earth, a bond that cannot be broken.

If the phone rang in the night, I asked Lois to answer. She was braver than I. She never thought of herself as brave. If she exclaimed "Oh my" or "Oh no," I interjected: "What happened? Who is it?" It was probably about a cat or a scratch on a child's knee or a broken demitasse. To me it was at least a broken bone, but hardly ever.

This is not a legacy I am proud to give my family. They have witnessed the struggle and the victory. They saw the perspiration and heard the gentle songs. They witnessed the tremble and fright and the calm and joy after the story. They know my fear and feel my faith. They have been part of the healing; they are compassionate and caring, but they are not burdened as their father. They have learned how to be well and to heal. A good family is a gift of God.

The circle around a nuclear family must not be a burden. For me the sacrament of Baptism marks the family line around all families, and we are one, together. There is help on every side. I am learning to find and receive this family care from all people. We all hear the voice: "What do you want?" and all answer: "Make me well."

O Master, from the mountainside
Make haste to heal these hearts of pain;
Among these restless throngs abide;
Oh, treat the city's streets again;
Till all the world shall learn your love,
And follow where your feet have trod;
Till glorious from your heav'n above,
Shall come the city of our God.[24]

For sixty years I have found ways to be creative, though anxious, in public gatherings. People still talk about it after fifty years: the time I unraveled one ball of yarn which hundreds held on to until they felt like one family, one people, one body. The yarn was then laid in the font. We felt as connected and intimate as a household; we talked about how baptism reminds us of being one family, all sisters and brothers. Baptism says it loudly: we are one nuclear family. We are not meant to be a restless throng. We are to be a peaceful family in a garden; we are preparing for the city of our God. This city with a garden makes me be well with wonder!

– An idea to practice –

The nuclear family is indeed a gift from God, but so is the larger family of the people of God. All people are people of God. We grow anxious when our family is in real or imagined danger. We can see threats both when there are threats and when there are not. And we long for the city of God and the family of God where threat is removed, danger gone, and joy abounds. You might memorize Revelation 21:2-5:

> And I saw the holy city, the new Jerusalem, coming down out of heaven from God. . . . And I heard a loud voice from the throne saying,
>
>> "See, the home of God is among mortals.
>> He will dwell with them as their God;
>> they will be his peoples,
>> and God himself will be with them;
>> he will wipe every tear from their eyes.
>> Death will be no more;
>> mourning and crying and pain will be no more,
>> for the first things have passed away."
>
> And the one who was seated on the throne said, "See, I am making all things new."

Then when anxiety over your family or the family of God arises, speak these words as a prayer until the anxiety begins to diminish. No matter what happens on earth, all will be well in the city of God.

- 23 -

Anxiety

Hope

Lord Jesus, think on me,
By anxious thoughts oppressed;
Let me your loving servant be
And taste your promised rest.[25]

The grandchildren love to help mother set the table and serve. Nathan age four is proud to help his father shopping in Home Depot and pounding nails. Evelyn in Tokyo anticipates my every need, as does her mother, and cares for me. Francis' best time is with his father, searching nature. I have not found them oppressed with anxious thoughts, as was I.

Lord Jesus, think on me,
By anxious thoughts oppressed;
Let me your loving servant be
And taste your promised rest.

A thousand what-ifs in my life have oppressed me and seldom happened. Each what-if that really happened has been a huge turning point in my life. These have been the great milestones in my years. I would not choose them. However, I cannot imagine my years without them. They have uncovered hope.

What if? What if? What if the tests turn out positive? Positive does not mean positive! What if the forecast is right and it does not rain for two weeks? What if something happens so I cannot work? What if we are late? What if we miss the flight? What if they had an accident? What if I do not get an invitation? What if they are caught in a blizzard? What if he loses his job? What if?

I have known highs and lows. Who has not? Something I fear happens; now what?

Farmers we knew watched the sky, felt the soil, dug to find the moisture line in the field, and followed a cloud from the far horizon. These were signs of hope. This brought hope in times of what-if!

We watched the earth holler for help! We saw waters roar through creeks and erase corn fields in one hour. We felt the hot dry wind carry swarms of locusts into green fields and new gardens. We heard them munching the fruit of the land. There was the refrain: what-if? Inside me and on every side I have learned to feel the refrain: what-if?

And then we planted trees. Mother planted vegetables once more. Father pruned broken branches. Farmers planted a crop that would grow fast in a short season. Next year there would be corn again; not this summer. Small signs of hope.

Mel died in the war, eighteen years old. This was not what the farm family had planned. They read the Bible and found the best words they could for the grave marker. The words were full of hope. It was the best they could do. They would read the sentence every week when they walked to the marble marker to weed and water.

Our parsonage yards were family memorials. Trees, bushes, lily ponds, rock gardens were to honor others and keep memories sacred. They were planted for funerals, baptisms, confirmation, weddings, anniversaries.

We chose fruit trees and planted them carefully. We dug the holes large enough to spread out the long roots, and watered them, believing they would grow, bloom and bear fruit. Our eyes were fixed on hope. The perennials lived through a bitter winter. The annuals grew miraculously from tiny seeds. We smelled the aroma from a distance. Our eyes and senses were fixed on hope.

The seeds planted in egg shells and standing on the kitchen window sill were not so much about growing a garden. The seed in the spring was about faith growing. The bantam chicks that hatched during holy week were not about the hen house but about the resurrection. Our hearts were fixed on hope.

The perennial on Mel's grave was about Easter. So was the reading on the marker of Mel's grave. The grass was fresh green. Our hearts were fixed on hope. The old songs of hope still ring true and are underscored by new sprouts and grass and buds and petunias. There is a sign even more assuring than springtime and cherry blossoms.

When he shall come with trumpet sound,
O may I then in him be found,
Clothed in his righteousness alone,
Redeemed to stand before the throne!

On Christ, the solid rock, I stand;
All other ground is sinking sand.[26]

While the what-ifs were building my child life, so was my love of these old hymns. We knew them by heart and every person in the sanctuary sang. We were one great country choir. I went to every funeral, and we believed. We hugged and cried and sang and prayed together. We grew cold under March umbrellas and under a green tent when it snowed. There was never enough space for we all came. I was a boy who believed. I knew the pictures of faith by heart, those in our houses and those in my mind. And yet I hunted for hope. I read hope, believe hope, see hope, and write hope. A funeral was never for real unless we sang:

When I draw this fleeting breath,
When mine eyelids close in death,
When I soar to worlds unknown,
See thee on thy judgment throne,
Rock of Ages, cleft for me,
Let me hide myself in thee.[27]

— An idea to practice —

It has been said (rightly to my mind) that ordinary people of faith learn their theology more from the liturgy and hymn lyrics than from preaching and teaching. That's also where hope and peace and comfort and joy come from—the music of the faithful. Buy yourself a hymnbook. On Sunday, if some lyric speaks to your heart or gives voice to your soul, go home and sing it all week until you have it memorized. In no time, you will have a storehouse of faith locked tight inside, ready to be sung in the face of anxiety.

Anxiety

Fear

Once there was a town that was frightened by a tornado.
No one was hurt, but they could have been.
A plague swept through the village and the hospital was filled.
Every family was most frightened. No one died, but they could have.
Catastrophes struck the people year after year.
No one was hurt or died, but they could have.
The town is no longer afraid of tornadoes and floods and plagues.
They fear something greater. They fear being afraid.
The people fear fear.

"We have nothing to fear but fear itself!" This refrain from the United States President's oval office still rings in my years. In time of war, a man in a wheel chair defined the worst fear—fear of fear.

I was fourteen. My fears were of my posture, school exams, right and wrong, truth, salvation, pimples, secret thoughts, death. This was the beginning of my Course 101 in fear.

All too soon the course became more difficult. Finally I found out that the course I was enrolled in was titled: Fear of fear. Not fear of death but the fear of fear of death. Then I discovered fear of fear of truth, fear of fear of pimples and posture and secret thoughts and salvation. Not fear of something realistic and tangible, but, fear of fear!

When did this insight by President Roosevelt become clear to me? In the writing of this book.

In those years when Roosevelt talked to the nation in Fireside Chats, I was building a world of fears. The polio shot was a big debate in our country school. If I get the shot, will I get polio? If I do not get the shot, will I get polio and need an iron lung? Will I catch pneumonia? Will a car hit us while we're walking to country school? Will my throat swell shut from diphtheria? What if I fell in the cistern? What if our house blew down? Will I get encephalitis like someone I saw in town? Am I getting a goiter? Those were some of my health issues.

Soon I was afraid only of fear itself. I tried to work out my fear in the dark at night, in church, in prayer, in drawing, in writing, in building tree houses, in climbing trees, in church, in fantasy. I was a boy of faith with great fears.

Fear of fear is an endless, fruitless, frightening whirlwind. It is like an arrhythmia attack whose chain must be broken by a shock to live. Anxiety can weigh like a yoke of iron. Jesus, what do you mean: "My yoke is easy and my burden is light"?

Though all the world with devils fill
and threaten to devour us,
we tremble not, we trust God's will:
they cannot overpow'r us.

Though Satan rant and rage,
in fiercest war engage,
this tyrant's doomed to fail;
God's judgment must prevail!
One little word shall triumph.[28]

Luther is my hero partly for his combat with *Anfechtung*, depression. It is reported that Luther felled the devil in the throwing of his ink well. Perhaps it was the ink in his writing that felled Satan's rage. I believe it was his writing "in the Word" that was his weapon.

For us it may also be a little word, a mantra, a refrain, a song, a verse, a poem, a wall hanging, a letter, an old voice from the past, a touch. Writing these pages has helped me face the foe, and confront my own tremble and doom and rage. We are not alone in this anxious journey; we sing: "the one of God's own choosing." What little word shall triumph? Here are some: Beloved—Touch—Trust—Amen—I Believe—Jesus—Child of God—Love.

If we in our own strength confide,
our striving turns to losing;
the righteous one fights by our side,
the one of God's own choosing.
You ask who this may be:
Christ Jesus, it is he,
the Lord of Hosts by name.
No other God we claim!
None else can win the battle.[29]

— An idea to practice —

Next to the name of Jesus, perhaps the strongest word in the universe is *love*. It has been said that "love conquers all." It's true—not romantic love, but that deep love which created, sustains, and moves the universe through time, God's love. John wrote it down: "There is no fear in love, but perfect love casts out fear. . ." (1 John 4:18), and "No one has ever seen God; if we love one another, God lives in us, and his love is perfected in us. . ." (1 John 4:12). When fear begins to move you along the path of anxiety, use these two verses to "triumph" over it. Let this "one little word" love stand between you and fear: know that you are loved, the beloved of God; know that in the grace of God you are called to be one of the great lovers of the world.

Notes

1 Simon Brown, *Lutheran Book of Worship*, Hymn 475 (Minneapolis: Augsburg Fortress Publishers, 1978).

2 Jan Struther, *Lutheran Book of Worship*, Hymn 469.

3 Charles Eliot, *Lutheran Book of Worship*, Hymn 296.

4 Herbert Brokering, *To Henry in Heaven: Reflections on the Loss of a Child* (Minneapolis: Augsburg Books, 2005), 26.

5 Edwin Hatch, *Lutheran Book of Worship*, Hymn 488.

6 Ibid.

7 Marjorie Jillson, *Lutheran Book of Worship*, Hymn 476.

8 Nicolaus L von Zinzendorf, *Lutheran Book of Worship*, Hymn 341.

9 Charles Eliot, *Lutheran Book of Worship*, Hymn 296

10 Ibid.

11 Washington Gladden, *Lutheran Book of Worship*, 492.

12 Adapted from: http://www.worldprayers.org/frameit.cgi?/archive/prayers/celebrations/may_you_be_filled_with.html

13 George Matheson, *Lutheran Book of Worship*, 324.

14 Paul Gerhardt, tr. John Kelly, *Lutheran Book of Worship,* 129.

15 Don Deines, *Forced About by God's Love.*

16 Lyrics & Music: Maewa Kaihan, Clement Scott, Dorothy Stewart, © 1913.

17 Matthias Claudius, *Lutheran Book of Worship*, Hymn 362.

18 Ibid.

19 Horatius Bonar, *Lutheran Book of Worship,* Hymn 497.

20 Maltbie Babcock, *Lutheran Book of Worship,* Hymn 554.

21 Laurence Houseman, *Lutheran Book of Worship,* Hymn 413.

22 Catherine Cameron, *Lutheran Book of Worship,* Hymn 463.

23 Thomas Pollock, *Lutheran Book of Worship*, Hymn 112.

24 Frank North, *Lutheran Book of Worship*, Hymn 429.

25 Sinesius of Cyrene, *Lutheran Book of Worship*, Hymn 309.

26 Edward Mote, *Lutheran Book of Worship*, Hymn 293.

27 Augustus Toplady, *Lutheran Book of Worship*, Hymn 327.

28 Martin Luther, *Evangelical Lutheran Worship*, Hymn 505.

29 Ibid.